Balancing pH Levels Deliciously

An Easy-to-Follow Acid-Alkaline Diet Cookbook for Beginners

Dr. Vivian Greene

Copyright © by Dr. Vivian Greene 2023.

Contents

Introduction

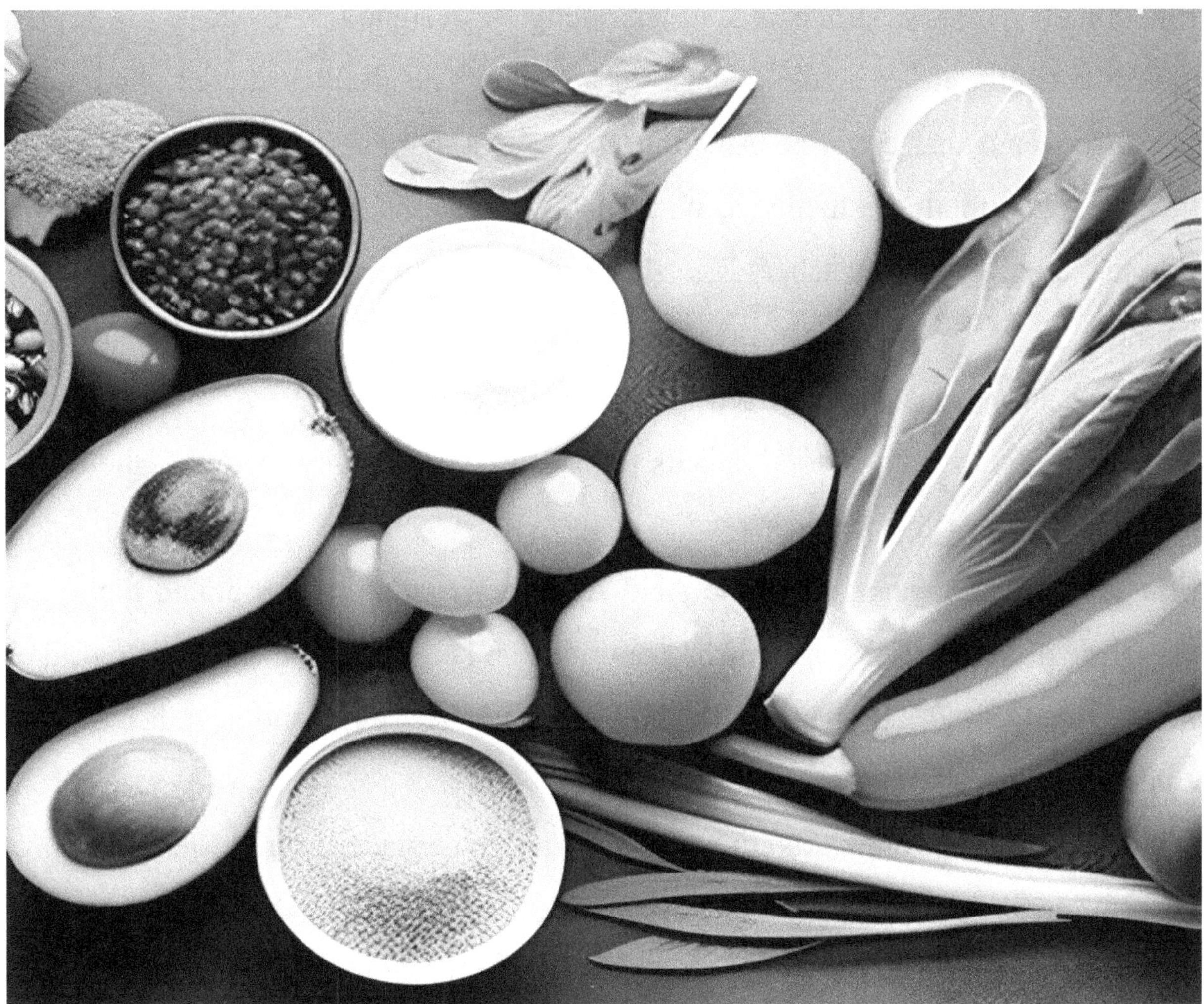

A remarkable collection of people who appeared to exude limitless energy and vigor lived in Alkalineville, a bustling town immersed in health and happiness. Their trick? The mysterious Acid-Alkaline Diet was a tried-and-true method of nutrition that had been handed down through the years. Many inquisitive people, including our main character Ella, were fascinated by this diet.

Ella, a vibrant young lady, discovered that she yearned for a life that was healthier and more stimulating. One day while she was strolling through the busy town market, destiny brought her to a worn cookbook that was concealed in a back room of an ancient bookstore. She enthusiastically flipped over its pages since it guaranteed a healthy and tasty diet.

Ella found a treasure trove of culinary delights designed to balance pH levels, improve health, and rekindle a sense of adventure inside the tattered parchment. She discovered that the Acid-Alkaline Diet was a symphony of wellbeing inside the body, a harmonic waltz between alkalizing and acidic foods.

Ella met a cast of wise teachers who shared their old knowledge and instructed her on how to make delectable breakfasts, filling lunches, healthful dinners, and seductive snacks as she immersed herself in this culinary journey. She discovered the magic of fresh, vivid food and its transformational ability to revive the mind, body, and spirit with each dish.

Ella accepted the principles of the Acid-Alkaline Diet and incorporated them into the fabric of her everyday life as she continued on her journey through the world of food. The outcome? A renewed vibrancy that lifted her spirits and gave her days an endless amount of energy.

Join us as we go through Alkalineville, a compelling place where tastes may cure, nourish, and rekindle the spark of life inside. You are invited to experience the wonder of healthful, scrumptious foods that feed your spirit and bring harmony to your complete body in "Balancing pH Levels Deliciously: An Easy-to-Follow Acid-Alkaline Diet Cookbook for Beginners". Get ready to uncover the genuine meaning of happiness and unleash your inner brightness.

Understanding the Acid-Alkaline Diet

Unlocking the keys to a peaceful and healthy existence requires understanding the Acid-Alkaline Diet. This dietary philosophy is based on the idea that the pH of the body determines its overall acid-alkaline balance. The basic idea is that we may promote optimum health and well-being by eating a diet that prioritizes alkalizing foods.

The interior milieu of the human body should be slightly alkaline for optimal performance. The pH scale is tipped toward acidity by the typical contemporary Western diet, which is typified by processed meals, meat, and sweet desserts. Numerous health problems, including weariness, inflammation, and reduced immunity, may result from this imbalance.

People who comprehend the Acid-Alkaline Diet are better equipped to choose the foods they eat with awareness and knowledge. Nutrient-dense, alkalizing foods including fresh fruits, leafy greens, vegetables, nuts, and seeds are prioritized in this diet. These whole foods provide a wealth of vitamins, minerals, and antioxidants that promote health and longevity in addition to helping to balance acidity.

The Acid-Alkaline Diet is a celebration of a variety of delectable foods rather than a restricted or trend-driven approach to balancing pH levels. It promotes a stronger connection between the body and the natural resources of the world by urging people to adopt a more holistic and thoughtful approach to eating.

Understanding the Acid-Alkaline Diet takes us on a journey to empowerment and renewal, where food turns becomes a source of pleasure and healing. A step and an alkalizing mouthful at a time, accepting this nutritional paradigm is an invitation to recover our health, energy, and happiness

What is the Acid-Alkaline Balance?

The foundational idea of the Acid-Alkaline Diet is the Acid-Alkaline Balance. This phrase describes the delicate balance between acidity and alkalinity inside the body. The pH scale, which goes from 0 to 14, with 7 being neutral, is used to quantify this equilibrium. A pH reading under 7 denotes acidity, whereas a reading above 7 denotes alkalinity.

Our bodies normally maintain a slightly alkaline pH level, usually between 7.35 and 7.45, when they are in perfect condition. This equilibrium, however, may be upset by elements like stress, unhealthful eating habits, and environmental toxins, which result in an acidic shift. The body attempts to counteract an increase in acidity by removing vital minerals like calcium and magnesium from tissues and bones, possibly weakening them over time.

For the various biological systems to work as they should, the acid-alkaline balance is essential. For optimum performance, several enzyme activities, cellular processes, and metabolic processes need certain pH values. The body may suffer from several health concerns such as weariness, inflammation, digestive disorders, and a weakened immune response when its pH level is too high.

The body's natural balance may be restored by understanding and maintaining the Acid-Alkaline Balance via the ingestion of alkalizing foods, which also helps to improve general well-being. Fresh produce, leafy greens, and other alkalizing foods should be prioritized if we want to aid the body's drive for health and longevity. The secret to unlocking the road to optimum health and energy is striking the proper balance between acidity and alkalinity.

Benefits of Balancing pH Levels

The advantages of maintaining a balanced pH level go well beyond maintaining good physical health; they also include a comprehensive feeling of well-being that affects all parts of our life. A multitude of benefits may be unlocked by preserving the body's ideal acid-alkaline balance.

pH equilibrium promotes greater vitality and higher energy levels. The body performs at its peak when the internal environment is balanced, allowing us to take on everyday difficulties with fresh vitality and excitement.

A pH that is in equilibrium helps the immune system perform better. The body strengthens its defense against sickness and disease by lowering excess acidity, which makes the environment less hospitable to germs.

Lowering inflammation, a typical precursor to many chronic illnesses, is a major benefit of maintaining pH balance. It promotes joint health, heals the body, and lowers the chance of illnesses including heart disease and arthritis.

The Acid-Alkaline Diet has been linked to enhanced nutritional absorption and improved digestion. The digestive system functions more effectively when pH levels are controlled, ensuring that vital nutrients are quickly absorbed and used by the body.

Balanced pH levels may support improved mental and emotional clarity, attention, and emotional stability. The mind feels lighter and more at peace when the body's acidity and inflammation are reduced, improving general cognitive performance and encouraging a positive view of life.

A wealth of health advantages are unlocked by adopting the practice of pH Level Balancing, leading the path to a renewed and peaceful living on the inside as well as the outside. We start along the path to a healthy, joy-filled existence by fueling our bodies with alkalizing foods, where well-being becomes the cornerstone on which we construct our hopes and desires.

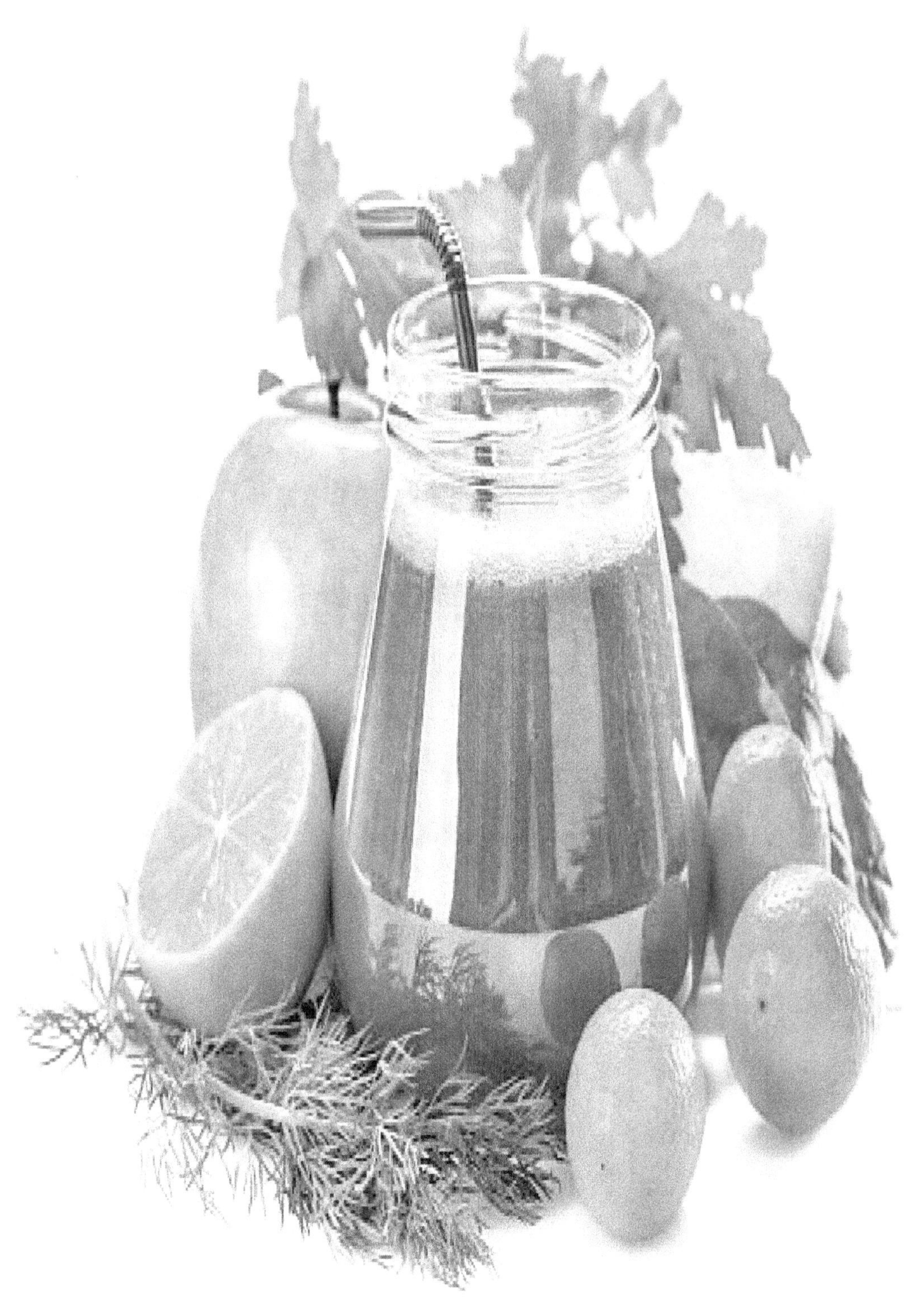

Foods to Embrace and Avoid

The Acid-Alkaline Diet's foods to embrace and avoid are essential for reaching and maintaining maximum health. People may make educated decisions to establish a harmonious internal environment by knowing which meals contribute to acidity and which ones have an alkalizing impact.

Including Foods that Alkalize:

Fresh Fruits: A wide variety of vibrant fresh fruits, such as apples, avocados, berries, citrus fruits, melons, and kiwis, are packed with important vitamins, minerals, and antioxidants. They not only maintain pH levels, but they also give off a natural energy boost and promote general well-being.

Dark leafy greens are nutritious powerhouses, including spinach, kale, Swiss chard, and collard greens. They support the alkalinity and detoxification of the body since they are rich in phytonutrients and chlorophyll.

Cruciferous Vegetables: Excellent sources of fiber, vitamins, and minerals include broccoli, cauliflower, Brussels sprouts, and cabbage. They promote a pH balance and help with digestion.

Almonds, chia seeds, flaxseeds, and pumpkin seeds are alkalizing and provide healthy fats, protein, and necessary elements.

Healthy Fats: Alkalizing avocado and coconut oils are healthful and make great substitutes for manufactured oils.

Herbal teas: In addition to being calming, herbal teas like chamomile, peppermint, and ginger also help the body become more alkaline.

Avoiding Foods That Form Acid:

Foods that have been processed and refined lack key nutrients and often contribute to acidity. Examples include white bread, sweet snacks, and prepared meals.

Meat and dairy: When digested by the body, animal items, particularly red meat, and dairy, tend to cause acidity.

Alcohol and Caffeine: Acidic drinks like coffee, tea, and alcohol may upset the pH equilibrium in the body.

Refined Sugar: Consuming too much-refined sugar, which is included in desserts and sugary drinks, may cause the body to become acidic.

Artificial sweeteners: In addition to being acidic, artificial sweeteners may also be harmful to your health.

Processed Fats: Due to their harmful effects on health, trans fats, and hydrogenated oils, which are included in fried and processed meals, should be avoided.

For the Acid-Alkaline Diet to work, it's crucial to comprehend the delicate balance between alkalizing and acid-forming foods. While consuming acid-forming meals on occasion is OK, maintaining a balanced pH and promoting general health requires a focus on complete, nutrient-dense foods that are alkalizing.

It's important to keep in mind that everyone's reactions to food may differ, therefore dietary limits and personal preferences should be taken into account while designing an acid-alkaline diet. People may start on a transforming path to optimum health, energy, and vitality by choosing their meals with mindfulness and intuition.

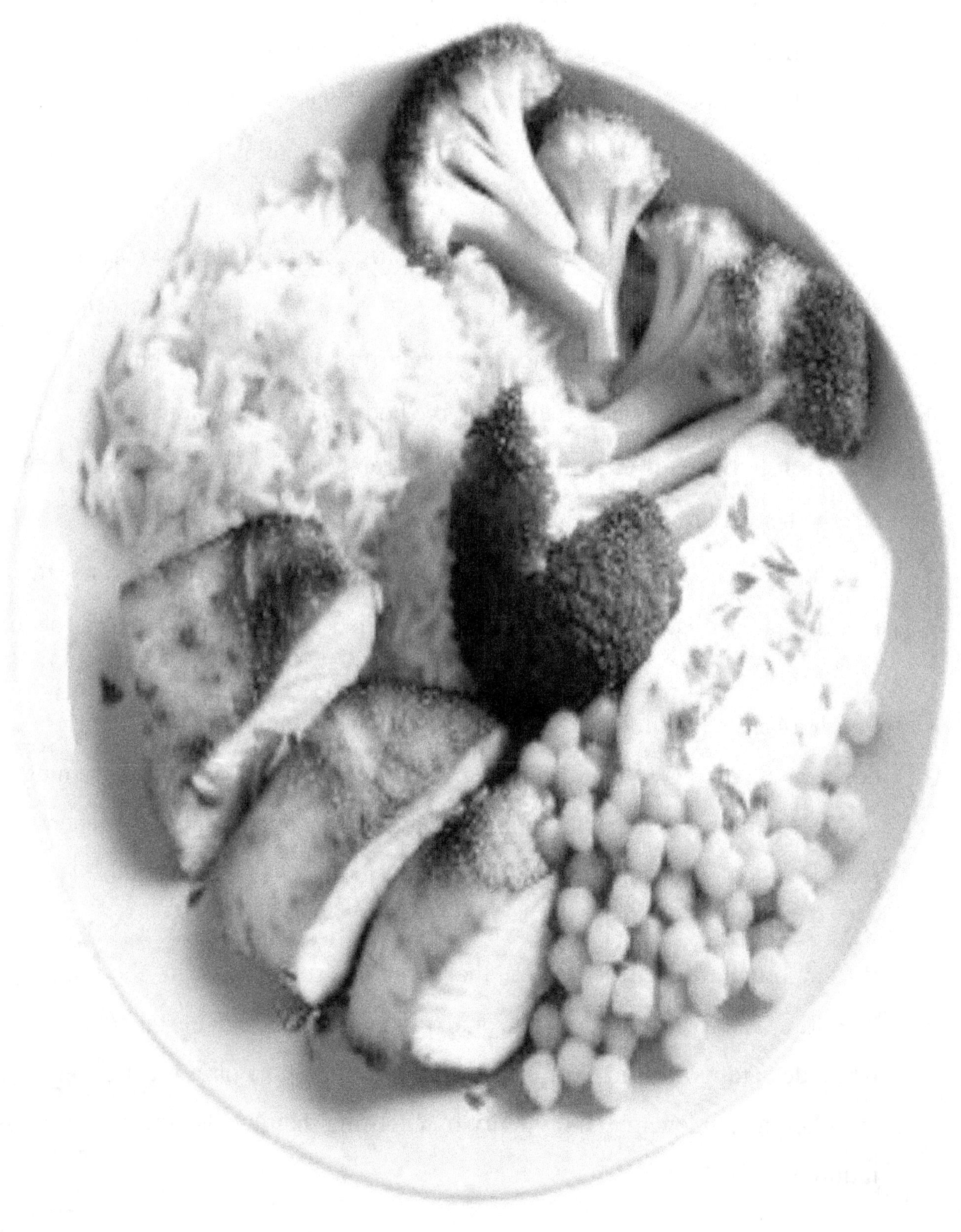

Chapter 1

ALKALIZING BREAKFASTS

Energizing Green Smoothie Bowl

Ingredients:

- 1 cup spinach (fresh or frozen)

- 1/2 ripe avocado

- 1 frozen banana

- 1/2 cup cucumber (peeled and chopped)

- 1/2 cup unsweetened almond milk (or any plant-based milk)

- 1 tablespoon chia seeds

- 1 teaspoon spirulina powder (optional, for an extra alkaline boost)

- Fresh fruit (such as berries, kiwi, or sliced apple) and nuts/seeds for toppings

Preparation:

1. In a blender, combine the spinach, avocado, frozen banana, cucumber, almond milk, chia seeds, and spirulina powder (if using).

2. Blend until smooth and creamy, adjusting the almond milk consistency if needed.

3. Pour the green smoothie into a bowl.

4. Top with your favorite fresh fruits and a sprinkle of nuts or seeds for added texture and nutrients.

Alkaline Information (per serving):

- Spinach: Alkalizing

- Avocado: Highly Alkalizing

- Banana: Moderately Alkalizing

- Cucumber: Alkalizing

- Almond Milk: Alkalizing

- Chia Seeds: Alkalizing

- Spirulina (optional): Highly Alkalizing

- Fresh fruits: Alkalizing

- Nuts/Seeds: Alkalizing

Superfood Almond Butter and Blueberry Smoothie Bowl

Ingredients:

- 1 cup fresh or frozen blueberries

- 1 tablespoon almond butter

- 1 cup kale leaves (stems removed)

- 1/2 cup unsweetened coconut water (or any plant-based milk)

- 1 tablespoon hemp seeds

- 1 teaspoon lemon juice

- Fresh blueberries and sliced almonds for toppings

Preparation:

1. In a blender, combine the blueberries, almond butter, kale leaves, coconut water (or plant-based milk), hemp seeds, and lemon juice.

2. Blend until smooth and creamy, adjusting the liquid consistency if needed.

3. Pour the vibrant smoothie into a bowl.

4. Top with fresh blueberries and sliced almonds for a delightful crunch and added alkaline goodness.

Alkaline Information (per serving):

- Blueberries: Alkalizing

- Almond Butter: Alkalizing

- Kale: Alkalizing

- Coconut Water: Alkalizing

- Hemp Seeds: Alkalizing

- Lemon Juice: Alkalizing

- Sliced Almonds: Alkalizing

Citrus Infused Chia Seed Pudding

Ingredients:

- 1/4 cup chia seeds

- 1 cup coconut milk (or any plant-based milk)

- 1 tablespoon maple syrup (optional, for sweetness)

- 1 teaspoon vanilla extract

- Zest of one organic lemon or lime

- Sliced oranges, grapefruits, or any citrus fruits for topping

Preparation:

1. In a bowl, mix the chia seeds, coconut milk, maple syrup (if using), vanilla extract, and citrus zest.

2. Stir well to combine, ensuring there are no clumps of chia seeds.

3. Let the mixture sit in the refrigerator overnight or for at least 4 hours to allow the chia seeds to gel and create a pudding-like consistency.

4. When ready to serve, spoon the citrus-infused chia seed pudding into a bowl.

5. Top with slices of your favorite alkalizing citrus fruits for a refreshing and nutritious morning treat.

Alkaline Information (per serving):

- Chia Seeds: Alkalizing

- Coconut Milk: Alkalizing

- Maple Syrup (optional): Acidic (use in moderation)

- Vanilla Extract: Alkalizing

- Citrus Zest: Alkalizing

- Citrus Fruits: Alkalizing

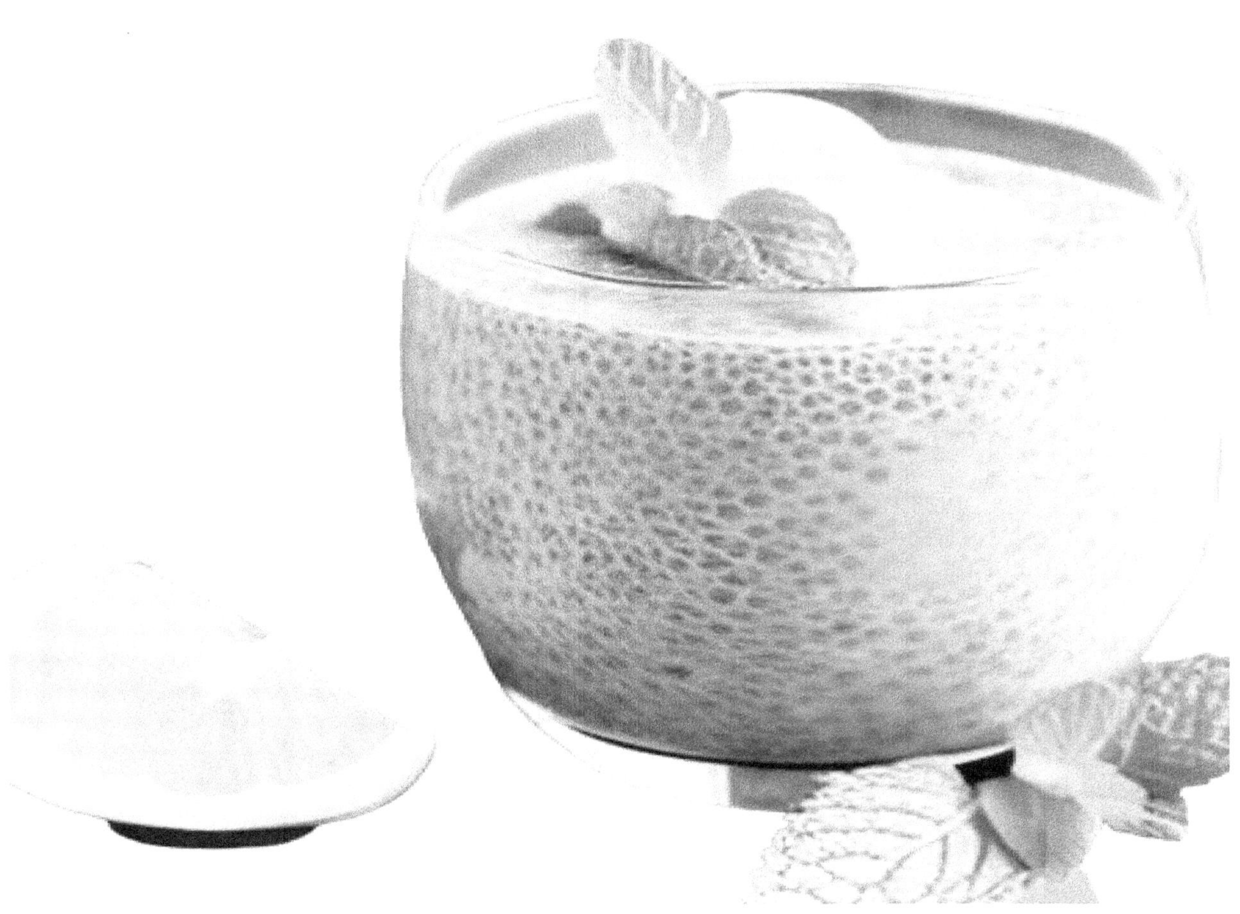

Quinoa and Veggie Breakfast Skillet

Ingredients:

1) 1 cup cooked quinoa

2) 1 tablespoon olive oil

3) 1 small onion, diced

4) 1 red bell pepper, diced

5) 1 zucchini, diced

6) 1 cup cherry tomatoes, halved

7) 2 cloves garlic, minced

8) 1 teaspoon dried oregano

9) Salt and pepper to taste

10) Fresh basil leaves for garnish

Preparation:

1) Heat olive oil in a large skillet over medium heat.

2) Add diced onion and sauté until translucent.

3) Add diced red bell pepper, zucchini, and cherry tomatoes to the skillet. Cook for 5-7 minutes, until the vegetables are tender but still crisp.

4) Stir in the minced garlic, dried oregano, salt, and pepper. Cook for another minute until the aroma fills the air.

5) Add the cooked quinoa to the skillet and toss everything together until well combined. Cook for an additional 2-3 minutes to allow the flavors to meld.

6) Remove from heat and garnish with fresh basil leaves for a burst of color and added freshness.

7) Serve this nutritious and alkalizing quinoa and veggie breakfast skillet warm and enjoy a wholesome start to your day.

Alkaline Information per Serving:

This alkalizing breakfast is a nutritional powerhouse, abundant in alkaline-forming ingredients. Quinoa, a gluten-free grain, provides a complete protein source, while the assortment of colorful vegetables offers an array of vitamins, minerals, and antioxidants. The alkaline-rich vegetables, including red bell peppers, zucchini, and tomatoes, help balance the body's pH levels, promoting overall well-being. The addition of olive oil contributes to the healthy fats required for absorption of fat-soluble vitamins. This delicious breakfast skillet not only satisfies your taste buds but also nourishes your body with alkaline goodness to kickstart your day on a positive note.

Citrus Infused Chia Seed Pudding

Ingredients:

1) 1/4 cup chia seeds

2) 1 cup almond milk (or any plant-based milk of your choice)

3) 1 tablespoon maple syrup (or sweetener of preference)

4) Zest of one organic orange

5) Zest of one organic lemon

6) 1/2 teaspoon pure vanilla extract

7) Fresh fruit (such as berries, sliced oranges, or kiwi) for topping

8) Optional: chopped nuts or coconut flakes for added crunch

Preparation:

1) In a mixing bowl, combine chia seeds, almond milk, maple syrup, orange zest, lemon zest, and vanilla extract. Stir well to ensure the chia seeds are evenly distributed.

2) Let the mixture sit for about 5 minutes, stirring occasionally to prevent clumps.

3) Cover the bowl with plastic wrap or a lid and refrigerate overnight, or for at least 4-6 hours, to allow the chia seeds to absorb the liquid and form a pudding-like consistency.

4) Before serving, give the pudding a good stir to ensure its evenly set. Add a splash of almond milk if you prefer a creamier texture.

5) Top the citrus-infused chia seed pudding with your favorite fresh fruits and optional toppings like chopped nuts or coconut flakes for added texture and flavor.

6) Enjoy this refreshing and alkalizing breakfast!

Nutrition Information (per serving):

- ❖ Calories: 230 kcal
- ❖ Total Fat: 11g
- ❖ Saturated Fat: 1g
- ❖ Sodium: 70mg
- ❖ Total Carbohydrates: 27g
- ❖ Dietary Fiber: 11g
- ❖ Sugars: 10g
- ❖ Protein: 6g
- ❖ Calcium: 380mg
- ❖ Iron: 3mg

❖ Vitamin C: 30mg

Creamy Lime and Coconut Chia Seed Pudding

Ingredients:

1) 1/4 cup chia seeds

2) 1 cup coconut milk (canned or homemade)

3) 1 tablespoon agave syrup (or sweetener of choice)

4) Zest of one organic lime

5) 1 tablespoon fresh lime juice

6) 1/4 cup diced fresh pineapple (or tropical fruits of your choice)

7) 2 tablespoons toasted coconut flakes for garnish

Preparation:

1) In a mixing bowl, combine chia seeds, coconut milk, agave syrup, lime zest, and fresh lime juice. Stir well to ensure the chia seeds are evenly distributed.

2) Allow the mixture to rest for 5 minutes, stirring occasionally to avoid clumps.

3) Cover the bowl with plastic wrap or a lid and refrigerate overnight or for at least 4-6 hours until the chia seeds have thickened and absorbed the liquid.

4) Before serving, stir the pudding to achieve a smooth and creamy consistency.

5) Top the lime and coconut chia seed pudding with diced fresh pineapple and toasted coconut flakes for a tropical twist.

6) Savor the delightful blend of flavors and the alkalizing goodness of this satisfying breakfast!

Nutrition Information (per serving):

- ❖ Calories: 280 kcal
- ❖ Total Fat: 18g
- ❖ Saturated Fat: 12g
- ❖ Sodium: 20mg
- ❖ Total Carbohydrates: 26g
- ❖ Dietary Fiber: 12g
- ❖ Sugars: 10g
- ❖ Protein: 6g
- ❖ Calcium: 250mg
- ❖ Iron: 3mg
- ❖ Vitamin C: 15mg

Zesty Grapefruit and Mint Chia Seed Pudding

Ingredients:

1) 1/4 cup chia seeds
2) 1 cup unsweetened grapefruit juice (freshly squeezed or store-bought)
3) 1 tablespoon honey (or sweetener of your choice)
4) Zest of one organic grapefruit
5) 1 tablespoon fresh mint leaves, finely chopped
6) Fresh grapefruit segments for topping
7) Fresh mint leaves for garnish

Preparation:

1) In a mixing bowl, combine chia seeds, grapefruit juice, honey, grapefruit zest, and chopped mint leaves. Stir thoroughly to evenly disperse the chia seeds.

2) Allow the mixture to sit for 5 minutes, occasionally stirring to prevent clumping.

3) Cover the bowl with plastic wrap or a lid and refrigerate overnight or for at least 4-6 hours until the chia seeds absorb the liquid and create a pudding-like texture.

4) Before serving, give the pudding a good stir to achieve a smooth consistency.

5) Top the zesty grapefruit and mint chia seed pudding with fresh grapefruit segments and a sprig of mint for an invigorating and refreshing breakfast.

6) Revel in the tangy citrus flavors and the alkalizing benefits of this delightful morning treat!

Nutrition Information (per serving):

- ❖ Calories: 190 kcal
- ❖ Total Fat: 8g
- ❖ Saturated Fat: 1g
- ❖ Sodium: 5mg
- ❖ Total Carbohydrates: 25g
- ❖ Dietary Fiber: 9g
- ❖ Sugars: 11g
- ❖ Protein: 5g
- ❖ Calcium: 180mg
- ❖ Iron: 2mg
- ❖ Vitamin C: 30mg

Fresh Fruit Salad with Almond Milk Yogurt

Ingredients:

1) 1 cup mixed fresh fruits (e.g., strawberries, blueberries, kiwi, and pineapple), chopped

2) 1/2 cup almond milk yogurt (unsweetened)

Preparation:

1) Wash and prepare the fresh fruits. Peel and chop the kiwi, dice the strawberries, halve the blueberries, and cut the pineapple into bite-sized pieces.

2) In a mixing bowl, combine all the chopped fruits to create a colorful and flavorful fruit salad.

3) Spoon the almond milk yogurt over the fresh fruit salad and gently toss until the fruits are evenly coated with the creamy yogurt.

Nutrition Information per Serving:

(Note: Nutrition information may vary depending on the specific fruits and brands of almond milk yogurt used.)

- ❖ Calories: Approximately 150-200 calories
- ❖ Protein: 4-6 grams
- ❖ Carbohydrates: 30-40 grams
- ❖ Fat: 3-5 grams
- ❖ Fiber: 5-7 grams

- ❖ Calcium: 150-200 mg
- ❖ Vitamin C: 50-70 mg
- ❖ Vitamin K: 30-40 mcg

Tropical Medley with Almond Milk Yogurt

Ingredients:

1) 1/2 cup diced mango
2) 1/2 cup diced papaya
3) 1/2 cup diced pineapple
4) 1/2 cup sliced banana
5) 1/2 cup almond milk yogurt (unsweetened)
6) 1 tablespoon shredded coconut (optional)

Preparation:

1) Peel and dice the mango, papaya, and pineapple into small chunks. Slice the banana.
2) In a mixing bowl, combine all the diced and sliced fruits to create a refreshing tropical medley.
3) Spoon the almond milk yogurt over the fruit mixture and gently toss until the fruits are coated with the creamy yogurt.
4) If desired, sprinkle shredded coconut on top for an extra tropical twist.

Nutrition Information per Serving:

(Note: Nutrition information may vary depending on the specific fruits and brands of almond milk yogurt used.)

- ❖ Calories: Approximately 180-220 calories
- ❖ Protein: 4-6 grams

- ❖ Carbohydrates: 35-45 grams
- ❖ Fat: 3-5 grams
- ❖ Fiber: 6-8 grams
- ❖ Calcium: 150-200 mg
- ❖ Vitamin C: 60-80 mg
- ❖ Vitamin A: 200-300 IU

Berry Blast Parfait with Almond Milk Yogurt

Ingredients:

1) 1 cup mixed berries (e.g., strawberries, blueberries, raspberries)

2) 1/2 cup almond milk yogurt (unsweetened)

3) 1/4 cup granola (gluten-free, if desired)

4) 1 tablespoon honey (optional, for added sweetness)

Preparation:

1) Rinse and drain the mixed berries. Slice the strawberries and keep the smaller berries whole.

2) In a serving glass or bowl, layer the almond milk yogurt, mixed berries, and granola to create a delightful parfait.

3) Drizzle honey over the top if a touch of sweetness is desired.

Nutrition Information per Serving:

(Note: Nutrition information may vary depending on the specific berries, granola, and brands of almond milk yogurt used.)

- ❖ Calories: Approximately 200-240 calories
- ❖ Protein: 5-7 grams

- ❖ Carbohydrates: 35-45 grams
- ❖ Fat: 4-6 grams
- ❖ Fiber: 7-9 grams
- ❖ Calcium: 150-200 mg
- ❖ Vitamin C: 40-60 mg
- ❖ Iron: 1-2 mg

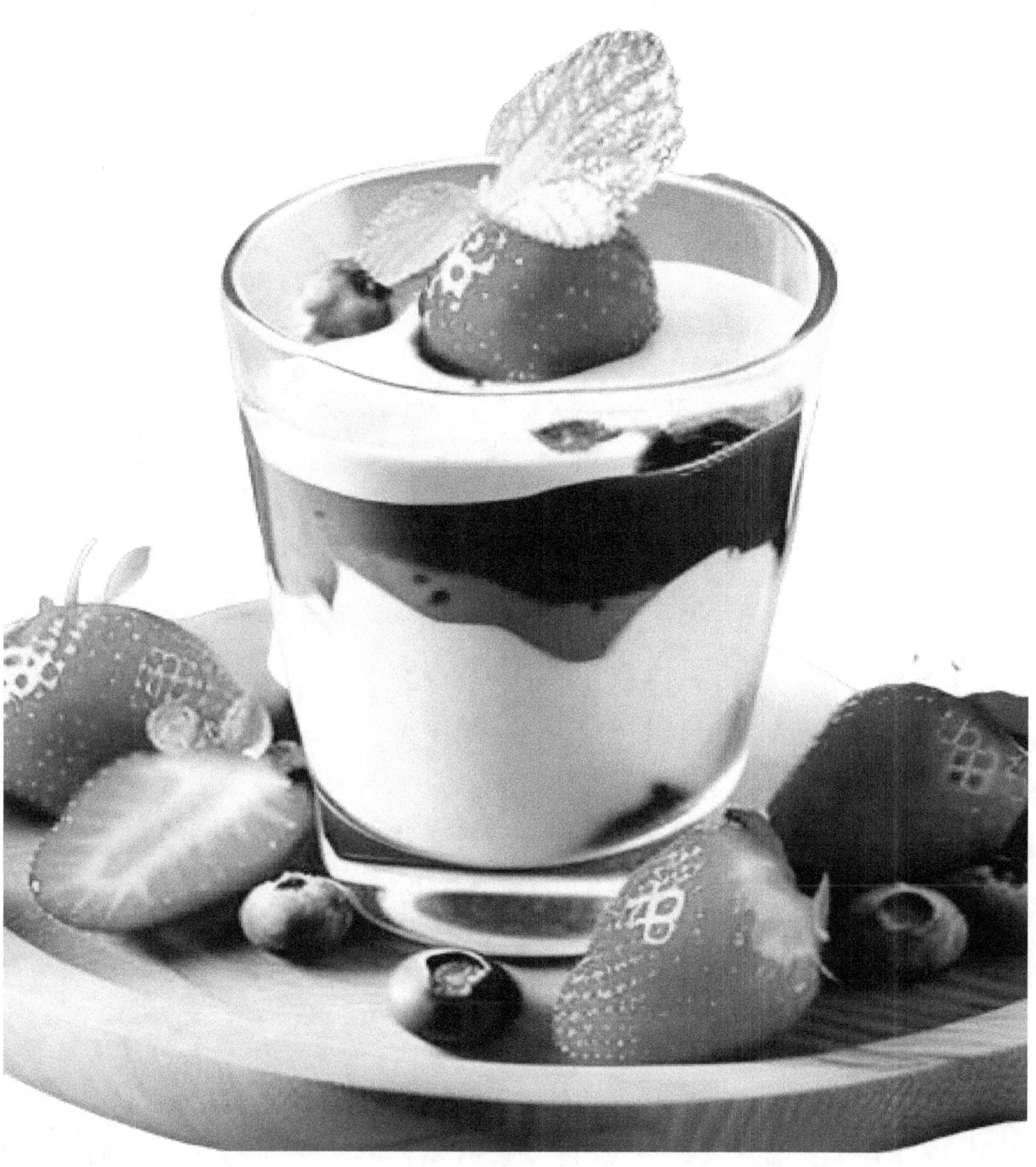

Chapter 2

NOURISHING LUNCHES

Grilled Portobello Mushrooms with Quinoa

Ingredients:

1) 2 large Portobello mushrooms

2) 1 cup quinoa

3) 2 tablespoons olive oil

4) 2 cloves garlic, minced

5) 1 teaspoon dried thyme

6) Salt and pepper to taste

7) 1 tablespoon balsamic vinegar

8) Fresh parsley for garnish

Preparation:

1) Preheat the grill to medium-high heat.

2) Clean the Portobello mushrooms and remove the stems. Using a spoon, gently scrape out the gills from the underside of the mushrooms to create more room for the quinoa filling.

3) In a saucepan, rinse the quinoa under cold water and drain. Add 2 cups of water and a pinch of salt, then bring to a boil. Reduce heat, cover, and simmer for about 15 minutes or until the quinoa is cooked and water is absorbed.

4) In a small bowl, mix together olive oil, minced garlic, dried thyme, salt, and pepper. Brush this mixture onto both sides of the Portobello mushrooms.

5) Grill the mushrooms for about 4-5 minutes per side or until they become tender and have grill marks.

6) Once the quinoa is cooked, fluff it with a fork and stir in the balsamic vinegar for extra flavor.

7) To serve, place the grilled Portobello mushrooms on a plate and stuff each mushroom cap generously with the cooked quinoa. Garnish with fresh parsley.

Nutrition Information (per serving):

- ❖ Calories: 350 kcal
- ❖ Total Fat: 12g
- ❖ Saturated Fat: 1.5g
- ❖ Cholesterol: 0mg
- ❖ Sodium: 15mg
- ❖ Total Carbohydrates: 50g
- ❖ Dietary Fiber: 8g
- ❖ Sugars: 2g
- ❖ Protein: 12g
- ❖ Vitamin D: 0mcg
- ❖ Calcium: 60mg
- ❖ Iron: 4mg
- ❖ Potassium: 750mg

Lemon Herb Baked Salmon with Steamed Veggies

Ingredients:

- 2 salmon fillets (wild-caught preferred)

- 1 lemon (sliced)

- Fresh herbs (such as dill, parsley, or thyme)

- 2 cups mixed vegetables (broccoli, cauliflower, carrots, etc.)

- 1 tablespoon olive oil

- Sea salt and black pepper to taste

Preparation:

1. Preheat the oven to 375°F (190°C). Line a baking sheet with parchment paper or lightly grease it to prevent sticking.

2. Place the salmon fillets on the prepared baking sheet. Season with sea salt and black pepper to taste.

3. Arrange the lemon slices and fresh herbs on top of the salmon fillets for added flavor.

4. Bake the salmon in the preheated oven for about 15-20 minutes or until the salmon is cooked through and flakes easily with a fork.

For the Steamed Veggies:

1. While the salmon is baking, prepare the mixed vegetables. Wash and cut them into bite-sized pieces.

2. In a steamer basket or a pot with a steamer insert, add water and bring it to a boil. Place the mixed vegetables in the steamer and cover with a lid.

3. Steam the vegetables for about 5-7 minutes or until they are tender-crisp. Be careful not to overcook them to retain their nutrients.

Nutrition Information (per serving):

- Calories: 350 kcal

- Protein: 25g

- Total Fat: 20g

  - Saturated Fat: 3.5g

  - Omega-3 Fatty Acids: 1.5g

- Carbohydrates: 15g

  - Dietary Fiber: 6g

  - Sugars: 4g

- Sodium: 150mg

This delightful Lemon Herb Baked Salmon with Steamed Veggies not only offers a burst of flavor but also provides a wealth of essential nutrients. Packed with omega-3 fatty acids, lean protein, and fiber-rich vegetables, this alkalizing lunch option supports a balanced pH and promotes overall well-being. Enjoy this nourishing meal as a satisfying midday treat that keeps you energized and revitalized throughout the day!

Alkalizing Nourishing Lunches:

Spinach and Avocado Salad with Toasted Almonds

Ingredients:

- 2 cups fresh spinach leaves

- 1 ripe avocado, diced

- 1/4 cup sliced cherry tomatoes

- 1/4 cup sliced cucumber

- 2 tablespoons toasted almonds

- 1 tablespoon extra-virgin olive oil

- 1 tablespoon balsamic vinegar

- 1 teaspoon lemon juice

- Pinch of sea salt and black pepper to taste

Preparation:

1. In a large mixing bowl, combine the fresh spinach leaves, diced avocado, sliced cherry tomatoes, and sliced cucumber.

2. In a separate small pan, toast the almonds over low heat until lightly golden and fragrant. Let them cool for a few minutes.

3. Add the toasted almonds to the salad mixture in the bowl.

4. In a small jar with a lid, combine the extra-virgin olive oil, balsamic vinegar, lemon juice, sea salt, and black pepper. Close the lid and shake vigorously to create the dressing.

5. Pour the dressing over the salad and gently toss all the ingredients together until they are evenly coated with the dressing.

Nutrition Information per Serving:

- Calories: 250 kcal

- Carbohydrates: 12g

- Protein: 6g

- Fat: 21g

- Fiber: 6g

- Vitamin C: 20% DV

- Vitamin K: 100% DV

- Folate: 25% DV

- Vitamin E: 15% DV

- Magnesium: 15% DV

This Spinach and Avocado Salad with Toasted Almonds is not only delicious and refreshing but also packed with essential nutrients. Spinach provides a rich source of vitamins K and C, while avocado adds healthy fats and fiber to keep you satisfied. The toasted almonds offer a delightful crunch and contribute to the salad's alkalizing properties. With its vibrant flavors and nourishing goodness, this salad is a perfect choice for a light yet satisfying alkalizing lunch that supports your overall well-being.

Lentil and Vegetable Stew

Ingredients:

1) 1 cup dried green or brown lentils, rinsed and drained
2) 1 tablespoon olive oil
3) 1 onion, finely chopped
4) 2 cloves garlic, minced
5) 2 carrots, peeled and diced
6) 2 celery stalks, diced
7) 1 red bell pepper, diced
8) 1 zucchini, diced
9) 1 can (14 oz) diced tomatoes
10) 4 cups vegetable broth
11) 1 teaspoon dried thyme
12) 1 teaspoon ground cumin
13) Salt and pepper to taste
14) Fresh parsley or cilantro for garnish (optional)

Preparation:

1) In a large pot, heat the olive oil over medium heat. Add the chopped onion and garlic, sautéing until they become translucent and fragrant.
2) Add the diced carrots, celery, red bell pepper, and zucchini to the pot. Cook for a few minutes until the vegetables start to soften.
3) Stir in the lentils, canned diced tomatoes, vegetable broth, dried thyme, and ground cumin. Season with salt and pepper to taste.
4) Bring the stew to a boil, then reduce the heat to a simmer. Cover the pot and let it cook for about 25-30 minutes or until the lentils are tender.
5) Adjust seasoning if needed and garnish with fresh parsley or cilantro before serving.

Nutrition Information per Serving:

- ❖ Calories: 230 kcal
- ❖ Protein: 12g
- ❖ Carbohydrates: 38g
- ❖ Fiber: 12g
- ❖ Fat: 4g
- ❖ Saturated Fat: 0.5g
- ❖ Sodium: 600mg
- ❖ Vitamin C: 35mg
- ❖ Iron: 4mg

This Lentil and Vegetable Stew is not only a flavorful and hearty lunch option but also an alkalizing powerhouse. Lentils are rich in protein and fiber, while the combination of colorful vegetables provides essential vitamins and minerals. The stew is packed with antioxidants and anti-inflammatory properties, promoting overall health and vitality. Enjoy this nourishing lunch to keep your body in an alkaline state and fuel your day with energy.

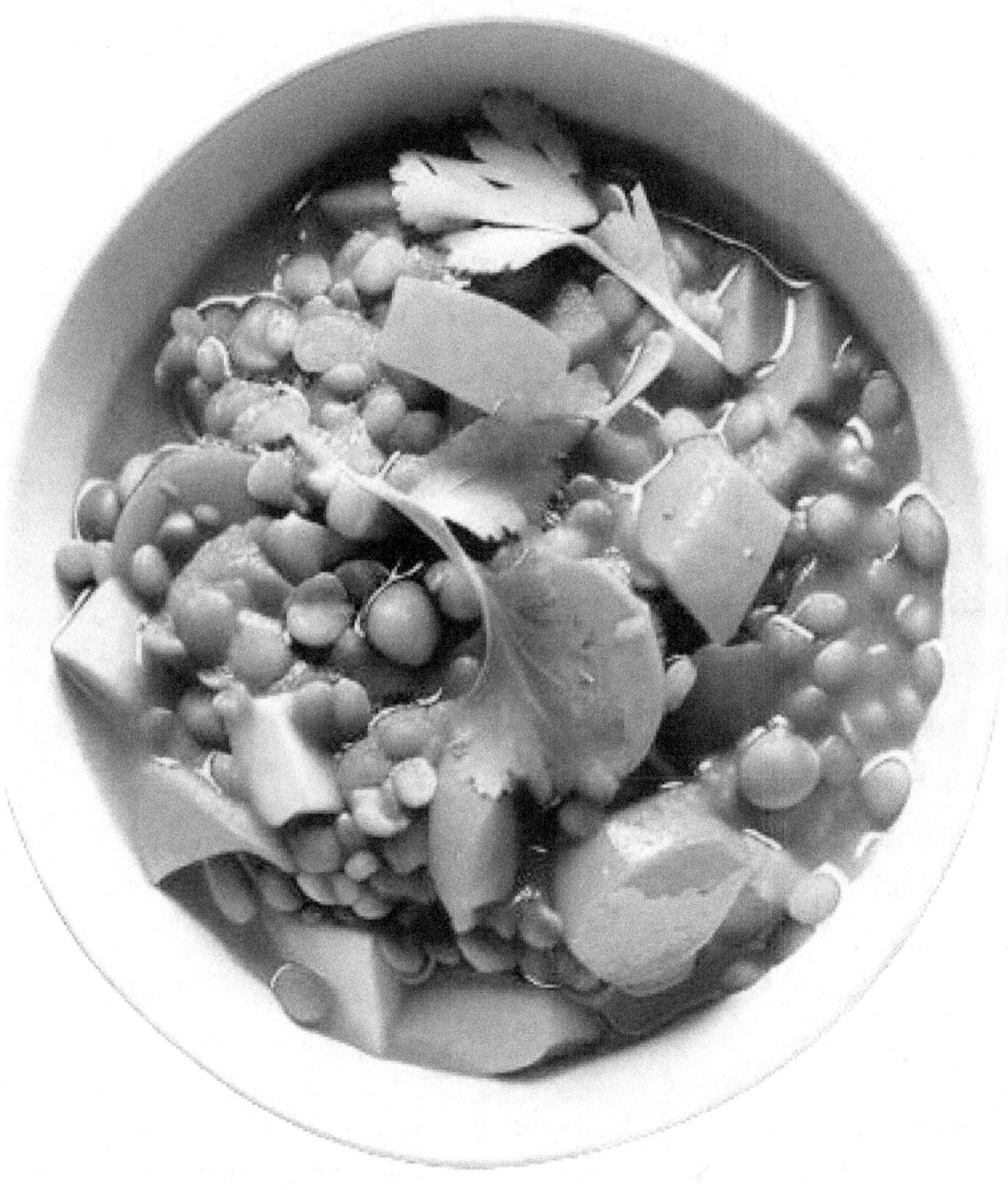

Chapter 3

WHOLESOME DINNERS

Zucchini Noodles with Creamy Avocado Sauce

Ingredients:

- 2 large zucchinis, spiralized into noodles

- 1 ripe avocado, peeled and pitted

- 1/4 cup fresh basil leaves

- 1/4 cup fresh parsley leaves

- 2 cloves garlic, minced

- 2 tablespoons freshly squeezed lemon juice

- 2 tablespoons extra-virgin olive oil

- Salt and pepper to taste

- Optional toppings: cherry tomatoes, pine nuts, grated Parmesan cheese

**Preparation: **

1. Prepare the zucchini noodles using a spiralizer, and set them aside in a colander to drain any excess moisture.

2. In a blender or food processor, combine the avocado, basil, parsley, minced garlic, lemon juice, and olive oil. Blend until smooth and creamy.

3. Season the avocado sauce with salt and pepper to taste, adjusting the flavors as desired.

4. In a large non-stick skillet over medium heat, add the zucchini noodles and cook for 2-3 minutes until they are just tender. Be careful not to overcook, as zucchini noodles can become mushy.

5. Remove the skillet from heat and add the creamy avocado sauce to the zucchini noodles. Toss gently until the noodles are evenly coated with the sauce.

6. Optionally, top the dish with halved cherry tomatoes, toasted pine nuts, and a sprinkle of grated Parmesan cheese for added flavor and texture.

7. Serve immediately as a delicious and nutritious dinner option.

Nutrition Information (per serving):

- Serving Size: 1/2 of the recipe (approximately 2 cups of zucchini noodles with sauce)

- Calories: 280 kcal

- Total Fat: 22g

- Saturated Fat: 3g

- Trans Fat: 0g

- Cholesterol: 0mg

- Sodium: 15mg

- Total Carbohydrates: 19g

- Dietary Fiber: 9g

- Sugars: 5g

- Protein: 5g

- Vitamin D: 0mcg

- Calcium: 60mg

- Iron: 2mg

- Potassium: 970mg

This Wholesome Dinner of Zucchini Noodles with Creamy Avocado Sauce offers a delightful combination of fresh flavors and satisfying creaminess without the need for heavy cream or pasta. It's a nutritious, low-carb option that is gluten-free, vegan, and full of essential vitamins and minerals. Enjoy the goodness of this light and refreshing meal, perfect for nourishing both body and soul.

Baked Stuffed Bell Peppers with Black Beans

Ingredients:

- 4 large bell peppers (any color of your choice)

- 1 cup cooked black beans (canned or pre-cooked)

- 1 cup cooked quinoa

- 1 cup diced tomatoes (canned or fresh)

- 1/2 cup diced onion

- 1/2 cup corn kernels (fresh, frozen, or canned)

- 1/2 cup chopped spinach or kale

- 2 cloves garlic, minced

- 1 teaspoon ground cumin

- 1 teaspoon chili powder

- 1/2 teaspoon paprika

- 1/2 teaspoon dried oregano

- Salt and pepper to taste

- 1 tablespoon olive oil

- 1/2 cup shredded cheddar or vegan cheese (optional, for topping)

Preparation:

1. Preheat your oven to 375°F (190°C).

2. Cut the tops off the bell peppers and remove the seeds and membranes. Rinse them under cold water and set them aside.

3. In a large skillet, heat the olive oil over medium heat. Add the diced onion and minced garlic and sauté until the onion becomes translucent.

4. Add the diced tomatoes, cooked black beans, corn kernels, chopped spinach or kale, ground cumin, chili powder, paprika, dried oregano, salt, and pepper to the skillet. Stir everything together and let it cook for about 5 minutes until the flavors combine.

5. Remove the skillet from the heat, and then stir in the cooked quinoa until it is well incorporated with the other ingredients.

6. Stuff each bell pepper with the mixture, pressing it down gently to fill all the spaces.

7. Place the stuffed bell peppers in a baking dish, and if desired, sprinkle shredded cheddar or vegan cheese on top of each pepper.

8. Cover the baking dish with aluminum foil and bake in the preheated oven for 25-30 minutes or until the peppers are tender.

9. Once baked, remove the foil and let them cool for a few minutes before serving.

__Nutrition Information (per serving - 1 stuffed bell pepper, without cheese):__

- Calories: 250 kcal

- Total Fat: 5g

- Saturated Fat: 1g

- Cholesterol: 0mg

- Sodium: 180mg

- Total Carbohydrates: 42g

- Dietary Fiber: 10g

- Sugars: 9g

- Protein: 11g

Note: The nutrition information provided is an approximate estimate and may vary based on the specific ingredients and quantities used. Adding cheese as a topping will increase the calorie and fat content.

Herbed Tofu Stir-Fry with Brown Rice

**Ingredients: **

- 1 cup firm tofu, cubed

- 2 cups cooked brown rice

- 1 cup broccoli florets

- 1 cup sliced bell peppers (assorted colors)

- 1 cup sliced carrots

- 1 tablespoon olive oil

- 2 cloves garlic, minced

- 1 tablespoon grated ginger

- 2 tablespoons low-sodium soy sauce (or tamari for gluten-free option)

- 1 tablespoon rice vinegar

- 1 tablespoon sesame oil

- 1 tablespoon fresh lemon juice

- 1 teaspoon dried oregano

- 1 teaspoon dried basil

- 1/2 teaspoon red pepper flakes (optional)

- Salt and pepper to taste

- Fresh cilantro or green onions for garnish

Preparation:

1. In a large skillet or wok, heat the olive oil over medium-high heat.

2. Add the cubed tofu and cook until it turns golden brown and crispy on all sides. Remove the tofu from the pan and set it aside.

3. In the same pan, add a little more oil if needed and sauté the minced garlic and grated ginger until fragrant.

4. Add the broccoli florets, sliced bell peppers, and sliced carrots to the pan. Stir-fry the vegetables for 3-4 minutes or until they are tender-crisp.

5. In a small bowl, mix the soy sauce, rice vinegar, sesame oil, lemon juice, dried oregano, dried basil, and red pepper flakes (if using).

6. Pour the sauce over the vegetables in the pan and stir to coat them evenly.

7. Add the cooked brown rice and tofu back into the pan. Toss everything together until the sauce is well distributed and the ingredients are heated through.

8. Season with salt and pepper to taste.

9. Serve the herbed tofu stir-fry over a bed of brown rice and garnish with fresh cilantro or green onions.

Nutrition Information (per serving):

- Calories: 380 kcal

- Protein: 15g

- Fat: 14g

- Carbohydrates: 49g

- Fiber: 7g

- Sugar: 5g

- Sodium: 440mg

Note: Nutrition information is approximate and may vary based on specific ingredients used.

Cauliflower Rice and Chickpea Curry

Ingredients:

- 1 medium cauliflower head

- 1 can (400g) chickpeas, drained and rinsed

- 1 large onion, finely chopped

- 2 cloves garlic, minced

- 1-inch ginger, grated

- 2 tablespoons curry powder

- 1 teaspoon ground cumin

- 1 teaspoon ground coriander

- 1 can (400ml) coconut milk

- 1 can (400g) diced tomatoes

- 2 tablespoons vegetable oil

- Salt and pepper to taste

- Fresh cilantro leaves for garnish

Preparation:

1. Begin by preparing the cauliflower rice. Wash the cauliflower head thoroughly and pat it dry. Remove the leaves and cut the florets into small pieces. Working in batches, pulse the cauliflower in a food processor until it resembles rice-like grains. Set the cauliflower rice aside.

2. In a large skillet or pan, heat the vegetable oil over medium heat. Add the chopped onion and cook until it becomes translucent, about 3-4 minutes.

3. Stir in the minced garlic and grated ginger, and cook for an additional minute until fragrant.

4. Add the curry powder, ground cumin, and ground coriander to the pan. Stir well to coat the onions, garlic, and ginger with the spices.

5. Pour in the coconut milk and diced tomatoes, and bring the mixture to a gentle simmer.

6. Add the cauliflower rice and chickpeas to the pan, stirring to combine all the ingredients.

7. Reduce the heat to low, cover the pan, and let the curry simmer for about 15-20 minutes, or until the cauliflower rice is tender and cooked to your desired texture.

8. Season the curry with salt and pepper to taste.

9. Serve the Cauliflower Rice and Chickpea Curry in individual bowls, garnished with fresh cilantro leaves for a burst of flavor and color.

Nutrition Information (per serving):

- Calories: 320 kcal

- Carbohydrates: 32g

- Protein: 9g

- Fat: 20g

- Saturated Fat: 16g

- Fiber: 9g

- Sugar: 6g

- Sodium: 680mg

This wholesome dinner of Cauliflower Rice and Chickpea Curry not only delights the taste buds with its aromatic spices but also nourishes the body with a generous serving of vegetables, plant-based protein, and healthy fats. Enjoy this flavorful and nutritious meal as a delightful addition to your Acid-Alkaline Diet journey!

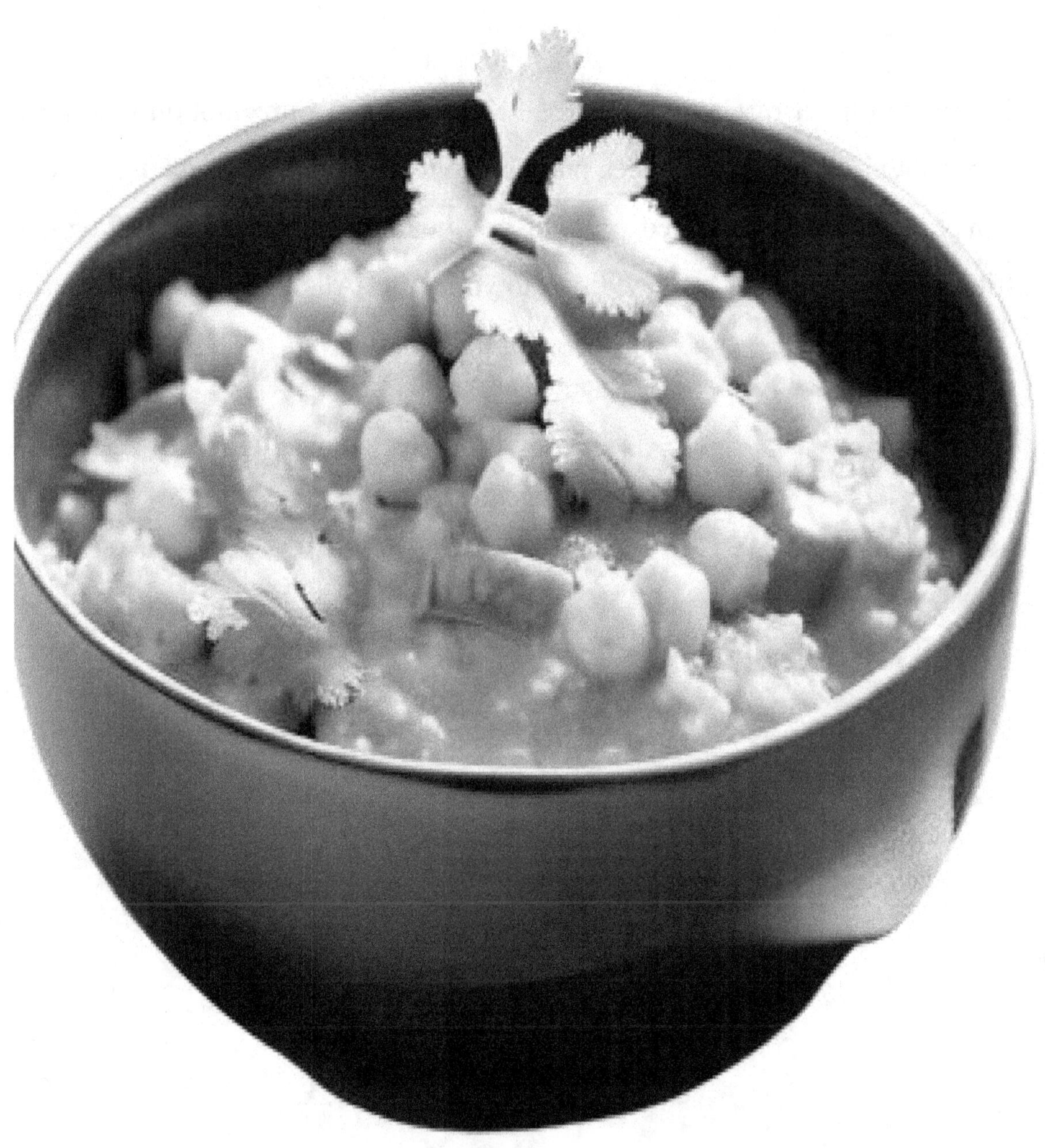

Chapter 4

DELECTABLE SNACKS AND SIDES

Cucumber and Hummus Bites

Ingredients:

- 1 large cucumber

- 1 cup hummus (store-bought or homemade)

- Fresh dill or parsley leaves for garnish (optional)

Preparation:

1. Wash the cucumber thoroughly under cold running water and pat it dry with a paper towel.

2. Slice the cucumber into thin rounds, about 1/4 inch (0.6 cm) thick.

3. Lay out the cucumber rounds on a serving platter or plate.

4. Using a teaspoon or a small piping bag, place a dollop of hummus on top of each cucumber round.

5. If desired, garnish each bite with a small dill or parsley leaf for an added touch of freshness and flavor.

6. Serve immediately or refrigerate until ready to enjoy.

Nutrition Information per Serving (approx. 4 cucumber and hummus bites):

- Calories: 50

- Total Fat: 2g

- Saturated Fat: 0.3g

- Trans Fat: 0g

- Cholesterol: 0mg

- Sodium: 130mg

- Total Carbohydrates: 6g

- Dietary Fiber: 2g

- Sugars: 1g

- Protein: 2g

- Vitamin D: 0mcg

- Calcium: 20mg

- Iron: 1mg

- Potassium: 152mg

Note: Nutrition information is approximate and may vary based on the specific brands of hummus used.

Alkaline Berry Blast Sorbet

Ingredients:

- 2 cups mixed berries (such as strawberries, blueberries, and raspberries)

- 1 ripe banana

- 1 tablespoon fresh lemon juice

- 1 tablespoon raw honey or maple syrup (optional, for added sweetness)

- 1/4 cup coconut water (or water, if preferred)

Preparation:

1. Wash the berries thoroughly and remove any stems or leaves.

2. Peel and slice the ripe banana into small chunks.

3. In a blender or food processor, combine the mixed berries, banana, fresh lemon juice, and raw honey or maple syrup (if using).

4. Blend the mixture until smooth, adding coconut water or water gradually until the desired sorbet consistency is achieved.

5. Taste and adjust sweetness by adding more honey or maple syrup if desired.

6. Pour the sorbet mixture into a shallow, freezer-safe container, and cover it with a lid or plastic wrap.

7. Freeze the sorbet for at least 3-4 hours or until it solidifies.

8. Serve the Alkaline Berry Blast Sorbet in chilled bowls or glasses and garnish with fresh berries or mint leaves, if desired.

Nutrition Information (per serving):

- Calories: 90 kcal
- Carbohydrates: 22g
- Fiber: 4g
- Sugars: 12g
- Fat: 0.5g
- Protein: 1g
- Vitamin C: 50mg (83% DV)
- Potassium: 180mg (5% DV)

Tropical Pineapple Lime Sorbet

Ingredients:

- 2 cups frozen pineapple chunks
- 1 ripe mango, peeled and pitted
- Zest and juice of 1 lime
- 2 tablespoons agave syrup or pure maple syrup (optional, for added sweetness)
- 1/4 cup coconut milk (canned, full-fat)

Preparation:

1. In a blender or food processor, combine the frozen pineapple chunks, ripe mango, lime zest, lime juice, and agave syrup or maple syrup (if using).

2. Blend the mixture until smooth, gradually adding coconut milk to achieve a creamy sorbet consistency.

3. Taste and adjust sweetness by adding more agave syrup or maple syrup if desired.

4. Transfer the Tropical Pineapple Lime Sorbet mixture into a shallow, freezer-safe container, and cover it with a lid or plastic wrap.

5. Freeze the sorbet for at least 3-4 hours or until it solidifies.

6. Serve the sorbet in chilled bowls or glasses, garnished with a lime slice or a sprinkle of shredded coconut, if desired.

Nutrition Information (per serving):

- Calories: 120 kcal

- Carbohydrates: 29g

- Fiber: 3g

- Sugars: 23g

- Fat: 1.5g

- Protein: 1g

- Vitamin C: 45mg (75% DV)

- Vitamin A: 2000 IU (40% DV)

Refreshing Watermelon Mint Sorbet

Ingredients:

- 4 cups seedless watermelon chunks (fresh or frozen)

- 1 tablespoon fresh lime juice

- 2-3 tablespoons fresh mint leaves

- 2 tablespoons agave syrup or honey (optional, for added sweetness)

Preparation:

1. If using fresh watermelon, remove the seeds and cut it into small chunks.

2. In a blender or food processor, combine the watermelon chunks, fresh lime juice, and fresh mint leaves.

3. Blend the mixture until smooth, taste, and add agave syrup or honey (if using) to enhance sweetness.

4. Pour the sorbet mixture into a shallow, freezer-safe container, and cover it with a lid or plastic wrap.

5. Freeze the sorbet for at least 3-4 hours or until it solidifies.

6. Serve the Refreshing Watermelon Mint Sorbet in chilled bowls or glasses and garnish with fresh mint leaves for a burst of flavor and color.

Nutrition Information (per serving):

- Calories: 60 kcal

- Carbohydrates: 15g

- Fiber: 1g

- Sugars: 13g

- Fat: 0g

- Protein: 1g

- Vitamin C: 15mg (25% DV)

- Potassium: 200mg (6% DV)

Enjoy these refreshing and alkaline fruit sorbet recipes guilt-free, knowing they not only satisfy your sweet cravings but also contribute to a balanced and nourishing diet.

Roasted Almonds with Turmeric and Sea Salt

Ingredients:

- 1 cup raw almonds

- 1 teaspoon ground turmeric

- 1/2 teaspoon sea salt

- 1 tablespoon olive oil

Preparation:

1. Preheat your oven to 350°F (175°C) and line a baking sheet with parchment paper.

2. In a mixing bowl, combine the raw almonds, ground turmeric, sea salt, and olive oil. Toss well to coat the almonds evenly with the seasoning.

3. Spread the seasoned almonds in a single layer on the prepared baking sheet.

4. Roast the almonds in the preheated oven for 12-15 minutes, or until they become golden and fragrant. Be sure to stir the almonds halfway through the roasting process to ensure even cooking.

5. Remove the baking sheet from the oven and let the roasted almonds cool completely before transferring them to an airtight container for storage.

Nutrition Information per Serving:

(Serving Size: 1 ounce, approximately 23 almonds)

- Calories: 160 kcal

- Total Fat: 14g

  - Saturated Fat: 1g

  - Trans Fat: 0g

- Sodium: 115mg

- Total Carbohydrates: 6g

  - Dietary Fiber: 3g

  - Sugars: 1g

- Protein: 6g

- Vitamin E: 7% DV (Daily Value)

- Magnesium: 20% DV

- Potassium: 4% DV

Note: The nutrition information is based on approximate values and may vary depending on the specific brands and quantities of ingredients used. Almonds are a nutritious snack rich in healthy fats, fiber, protein, and essential nutrients. The addition of turmeric not only imparts a warm, earthy flavor but also contributes to the health benefits of the dish with its anti-inflammatory properties. Enjoy these roasted almonds as a delicious and nourishing snack, or add them to salads, yogurt, or your favorite dishes for an extra boost of flavor and nutrition.

Guacamole and Veggie Sticks

Ingredients:

- 2 ripe avocados

- 1 small red onion, finely diced

- 1-2 cloves of garlic, minced

- 1 ripe tomato, diced

- 1 jalapeno or serrano pepper, seeded and minced (optional, for a spicy kick)

- Juice of 1 lime

- 2 tablespoons fresh cilantro, chopped

- Salt and pepper to taste

- Assorted veggie sticks (carrots, cucumber, bell peppers, celery, etc.) for dipping

Preparation:

1. Cut the avocados in half, remove the pits, and scoop the flesh into a mixing bowl.

2. Use a fork to mash the avocados to your desired consistency (smooth or chunky).

3. Add the finely diced red onion, minced garlic, diced tomato, and minced jalapeno/serrano pepper (if using) to the mashed avocados.

4. Squeeze the lime juice over the mixture and stir to combine.

5. Fold in the chopped cilantro and season with salt and pepper to taste.

6. Transfer the guacamole to a serving bowl and cover it with plastic wrap, ensuring it touches the surface of the guacamole to prevent browning.

7. Chill the guacamole in the refrigerator for at least 30 minutes to allow the flavors to meld.

8. Prepare the veggie sticks by cutting carrots, cucumber, bell peppers, celery, or any other preferred veggies into thin strips for dipping.

Nutrition Information (per serving):

(Note: Serving size may vary based on individual preferences.)

- Calories: 120

- Total Fat: 9g

  - Saturated Fat: 1.5g

  - Trans Fat: 0g

- Cholesterol: 0mg

- Sodium: 10mg

- Total Carbohydrates: 10g

  - Dietary Fiber: 7g

  - Sugars: 2g

- Protein: 2g

Guacamole and Veggie Sticks make for a wholesome and delicious appetizer, snack, or party treat. The creamy and flavorful guacamole pairs perfectly with an assortment of fresh, crunchy veggie sticks. This nutrient-rich snack is loaded with heart-healthy monounsaturated fats from avocados, providing a good source of fiber and essential vitamins. The addition of fresh vegetables adds extra nutrients, making it a guilt-free and satisfying option for any occasion. Enjoy this tasty and healthful dish with friends and family, knowing you're nourishing your body while indulging in a delightful culinary experience!

Chapter 5

SWEET AND ALKALINE TREATS

Sweet and Alkaline Treats: Coconut and Berry Chia Seed Popsicles

Ingredients:

- 1 cup coconut milk

- 1 cup mixed berries (strawberries, blueberries, raspberries)

- 2 tablespoons chia seeds

- 1 tablespoon agave syrup or maple syrup (optional, for added sweetness)

- Popsicle molds and sticks

Preparation:

1. In a blender, combine the coconut milk, mixed berries, and agave syrup (if using). Blend until smooth and well combined.

2. Pour the berry coconut mixture into a mixing bowl and stir in the chia seeds. Mix thoroughly to evenly distribute the chia seeds.

3. Allow the mixture to sit for about 5 minutes, allowing the chia seeds to soak up some of the liquid and thicken the mixture slightly.

4. After the mixture has thickened, pour it into popsicle molds, leaving a little space at the top to accommodate the sticks.

5. Insert popsicle sticks into each mold and gently tap the molds on the counter to remove any air bubbles.

6. Place the molds in the freezer and let them freeze for at least 4-6 hours or until completely solid.

<u>Nutrition Information (per serving):</u>

- Serving Size: 1 popsicle

- Calories: 80

- Total Fat: 4.5g

- Saturated Fat: 3g

- Trans Fat: 0g

- Cholesterol: 0mg

- Sodium: 5mg

- Total Carbohydrates: 8g

- Dietary Fiber: 3g

- Sugars: 3g

- Protein: 2g

Enjoy these delightful Coconut and Berry Chia Seed Popsicles guilt-free! These refreshing treats are not only a delicious way to beat the heat but also packed with nutrients. The combination of coconut milk, mixed berries, and chia seeds offers a perfect balance of flavors and textures. The chia seeds not only add a subtle crunch but also provide an abundance of healthy omega-3 fatty acids, fiber, and antioxidants. Plus, with no added refined sugar, these popsicles are a wholesome and nourishing treat for the entire family. Whether it's a sunny afternoon or a dessert craving strikes, these popsicles are sure to satisfy your sweet tooth while supporting your alkaline lifestyle. So go ahead, indulge in the goodness of Coconut and Berry Chia Seed Popsicles!

Sweet and Alkaline Treats: Almond Flour Banana Bread

Ingredients:

- 2 ripe bananas, mashed
- 3 large eggs
- 1/4 cup coconut oil, melted
- 1/4 cup pure maple syrup
- 1 teaspoon pure vanilla extract
- 2 cups almond flour
- 1 teaspoon baking powder
- 1/2 teaspoon baking soda
- 1/4 teaspoon salt
- 1/2 teaspoon ground cinnamon
- Optional toppings: sliced bananas, chopped almonds, or a drizzle of maple syrup

Preparation:

1. Preheat your oven to 350°F (175°C). Grease a standard 9x5-inch loaf pan with coconut oil or line it with parchment paper for easy removal.

2. In a large mixing bowl, combine the mashed bananas, eggs, melted coconut oil, maple syrup, and vanilla extract. Whisk the wet ingredients until well combined.

3. In a separate bowl, mix the almond flour, baking powder, baking soda, salt, and ground cinnamon.

4. Gradually add the dry ingredients to the wet ingredients, stirring until a smooth batter forms.

5. Pour the banana bread batter into the prepared loaf pan and spread it evenly.

6. If desired, decorate the top with sliced bananas, chopped almonds, or a light drizzle of maple syrup for added sweetness.

7. Bake in the preheated oven for 45 to 50 minutes or until a toothpick inserted in the center comes out clean.

8. Once done, remove the banana bread from the oven and let it cool in the pan for about 10 minutes. Then transfer it to a wire rack to cool completely before slicing.

Nutrition Information per Serving (serves 10):

- Calories: 210 kcal
- Total Fat: 15g
  - Saturated Fat: 6g
- Cholesterol: 56mg
- Sodium: 148mg
- Total Carbohydrates: 15g
  - Dietary Fiber: 3g
  - Sugars: 8g
- Protein: 6g

Indulge in this delicious and wholesome Almond Flour Banana Bread, a guilt-free sweet treat that's not only satisfying but also supports your body's alkaline balance. Enjoy it as a nourishing breakfast or a delightful snack, knowing that each bite contributes to your overall well-being!

Baked Apples with Cinnamon and Maple Syrup

Ingredients:

- 4 medium-sized apples (any sweet variety like Honeycrisp or Gala)

- 2 tablespoons pure maple syrup

- 1 teaspoon ground cinnamon

- 1 tablespoon coconut oil (or melted butter, if preferred)

- A pinch of sea salt

- Optional toppings: Chopped nuts, raisins, or a drizzle of almond butter

Preparation:

1. Preheat your oven to 375°F (190°C) and line a baking dish with parchment paper or lightly grease it with coconut oil.

2. Wash the apples thoroughly and pat them dry. Using an apple corer or a small knife, carefully remove the core and seeds, creating a well in the center of each apple.

3. In a small bowl, mix the maple syrup, ground cinnamon, coconut oil (or melted butter), and a pinch of sea salt until well combined.

4. Place the cored apples in the prepared baking dish, and evenly spoon the cinnamon-maple mixture into the center of each apple, allowing it to overflow slightly onto the sides.

5. For added flavor and texture, you can sprinkle chopped nuts or raisins on top of the apples at this stage.

6. Bake the apples in the preheated oven for 25-30 minutes or until they become tender and slightly caramelized.

7. Remove the baked apples from the oven and let them cool for a few minutes before serving.

Nutrition Information (per serving, based on 1 medium-sized apple):

- Calories: 150 kcal

- Total Fat: 3g

  - Saturated Fat: 2g

  - Trans Fat: 0g

- Cholesterol: 0mg

- Sodium: 30mg

- Total Carbohydrates: 32g

  - Dietary Fiber: 5g

  - Sugars: 24g

- Protein: 1g

- Vitamin D: 0mcg

- Calcium: 40mg

- Iron: 1mg

- Potassium: 220mg

Indulge in the warm, aromatic delight of these Baked Apples with Cinnamon and Maple Syrup. This sweet treat not only satisfies your cravings but also aligns with the principles of the Alkaline Diet. The natural sweetness of the apples, coupled with the warm notes of cinnamon and maple syrup, creates a delectable combination that's sure to enchant your taste buds. Enjoy these nutritious, guilt-free delights as a wholesome dessert, breakfast accompaniment, or a delightful snack any time of the day!

Raw Chocolate Avocado Mousse

Ingredients:

- 2 ripe avocados

- 1/4 cup raw cacao powder

- 1/4 cup pure maple syrup or agave nectar

- 1 tsp vanilla extract

- Pinch of sea salt

- Optional toppings: fresh berries, sliced almonds, or cacao nibs

Preparation:

1. Cut the avocados in half, remove the pit, and scoop out the flesh into a blender or food processor.

2. Add the raw cacao powder, pure maple syrup or agave nectar, vanilla extract, and a pinch of sea salt to the blender.

3. Blend the ingredients on high until you achieve a smooth and creamy texture. You may need to stop and scrape down the sides of the blender with a spatula to ensure all ingredients are fully incorporated.

4. Taste the mousse and adjust the sweetness to your preference by adding more maple syrup or agave if desired.

5. Once the mousse is smooth and velvety, transfer it to individual serving dishes or a large bowl.

6. Refrigerate the mousse for at least 30 minutes to allow the flavors to meld and the texture to firm up.

7. When ready to serve, garnish with fresh berries, sliced almonds, or cacao nibs for added texture and visual appeal.

Nutrition Information per Serving (Serves 4):

- Calories: 180 kcal
- Total Fat: 12g
  - Saturated Fat: 2g
  - Trans Fat: 0g
- Cholesterol: 0mg
- Sodium: 50mg
- Total Carbohydrates: 20g
  - Dietary Fiber: 7g
  - Sugars: 11g
- Protein: 3g

Note: This raw chocolate avocado mousse is not only a delectable treat but also a guilt-free indulgence. Avocado's natural creaminess combined with the richness of raw cacao makes for a luscious dessert that's packed with nutrients and health benefits. Avocados offer heart-healthy monounsaturated fats, fiber, and essential vitamins and minerals. Raw cacao is a potent source of antioxidants and mood-enhancing compounds. With a delightful balance of flavors and textures, this sweet and alkaline treat is sure to please your taste buds while nourishing your body from the inside out. Enjoy it as a satisfying dessert or a wholesome snack any time you crave a touch of decadence.

Chapter 6

CREATING BALANCED MEALS AND MENUS

Portion Control and Meal Planning Tips

Managing portions:

A key component of maintaining a balanced and nutritious diet is portion management. It entails being aware of how much food we eat at each meal and snack. We may avoid overeating, unneeded weight gain, and poor digestion by exercising portion control. Using smaller plates and bowls to give the appearance of a full plate while eating less is a useful tactic. Another piece of advice is to pay attention to our bodies hunger signals and stop eating when we are full rather than when we are overstuffed. Additionally, portioning meals and snacks beforehand helps prevent mindless eating and helps us stay on track with our dietary objectives. We may enjoy our favorite meals in moderation while enhancing our general health by making portion management a lifelong practice.

Tips for Meal Planning:

Making healthy eating more feasible and helping us remain on track with our nutritional goals is meal planning. Start by designating a certain time each week to plan your meals and make an appropriate shopping list. To guarantee a well-rounded diet, include a range of nutrient-dense foods such as fruits, vegetables, lean meats, and whole grains. Batch cooking or meal planning may save time and lessen the temptation to choose unhealthy fast food choices. To make meals interesting and delightful, try out various dishes and tastes. Planning your snacks is equally important since it helps you avoid making rash, unhealthy decisions. Last but not least, be adaptable and willing to make changes depending on your preferences and timetable. We may maintain our nutritional targets, cultivate a healthy relationship with food, and enjoy the advantages of a well-planned gastronomic adventure by preparing our meals mindfully.

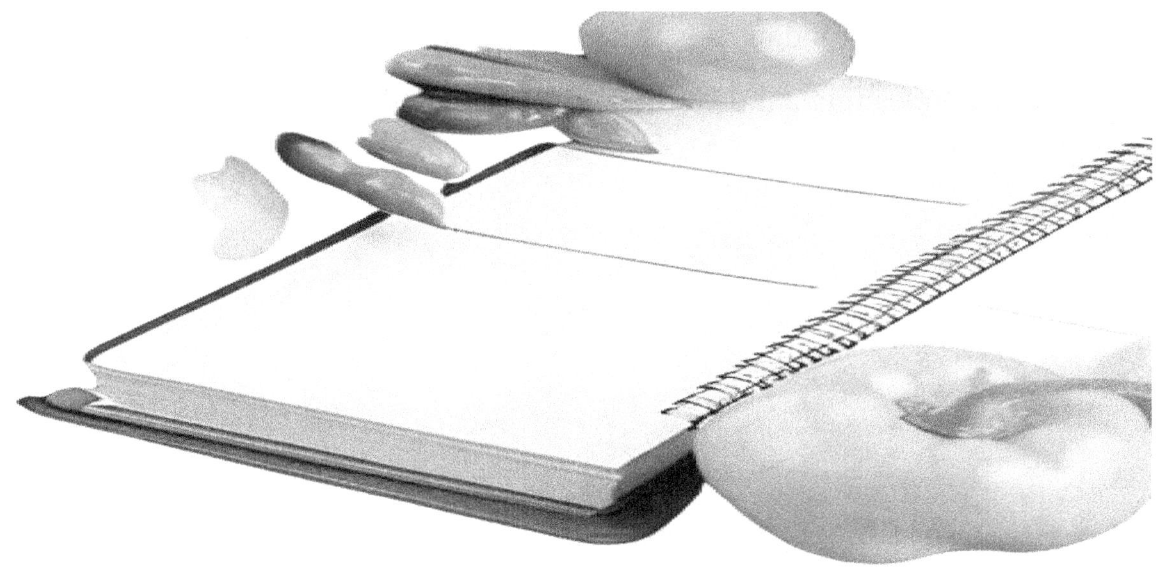

Balancing Protein and Plant-Based Foods

The Acid-Alkaline Diet promotes general health and vigor by balancing protein and plant-based meals. Including a variety of plant-based protein sources guarantees that people get the critical amino acids, vitamins, and minerals they need while keeping their bodies in an alkaline condition.

Legumes (such as lentils, chickpeas, and beans), tofu, tempeh, quinoa, almonds, and seeds are examples of plant-based protein sources that deliver a variety of nutrients without the acidic load sometimes associated with animal-based proteins. In addition to being superior sources of protein, they are also high in fiber, antioxidants, and good fats.

People may make nutritious, delicious meals that feed the body and encourage an alkaline pH by mixing different plant-based foods. Adopting this protein philosophy is advantageous for one's health as well as for the environment and the welfare of animals. Finding the ideal protein-to-plant food ratio is a simple yet effective step in leading a more sustainable and health-conscious lifestyle.

Combining Alkaline Ingredients for Maximum Benefit

The secret to optimizing the advantages of the Acid-Alkaline Diet is to carefully combine alkaline components. People may improve vitamin absorption, increase energy levels, and advance general wellbeing by preparing well-balanced meals.

Combining alkalizing fruits and vegetables with plant-based protein sources like beans, lentils, or tofu is one strategy. This mixture keeps the body's pH level alkaline while providing a full and healthy meal.

Additionally, combining citrus fruits and leafy greens in the same meal improves iron absorption because the citrus fruits' vitamin C content. This potent combination helps to maintain an alkaline pH while also enhancing immunity.

Alkalizing greens and healthy fats like avocado or almonds help the body absorb fat-soluble vitamins and maintain a healthy digestive tract.

Last but not least, adding taste to foods without sacrificing their alkaline nature is possible by using alkaline herbs and spices like basil, oregano, and turmeric.

People may make savory, filling meals that enhance health and energy while preserving the body's natural equilibrium by expertly blending alkaline components.

Conclusion

The Acid-Alkaline Lifestyle is a transforming path to optimum health and energy, to sum up. We may unleash the potential for greater well-being and vitality by knowing the delicate balance of pH levels and making deliberate dietary choices.

We have learned how to use alkalizing products to nurture the body and the spirit along this culinary journey. The Acid-Alkaline Diet provides a delicious variety of tastes that heal and inspire, from invigorating green smoothie bowls to delicious raw chocolate avocado mousse.

The Acid-Alkaline Lifestyle includes a comprehensive approach to well-being that goes beyond the kitchen, encouraging mindful eating, regular exercise, and stress reduction. It inspires us to rediscover the abundance of the Earth and refuel with natural resources.

We have a revitalized feeling of vigor and an awakened spirit when we adopt this way of life. The Acid-Alkaline Lifestyle gives us the power to take control of our health while promoting our body's natural capacity for healing and growth.

So let's start on this amazing trip, enjoying every healthy mouthful and the vivacious energy coursing through our veins. By adopting the Acid-Alkaline Lifestyle, we take control of our health, fostering inner harmony and shining our best selves out into the world. Let's commemorate the mystique of food, the virtue of balance, and the pleasure of living in harmony with nature's guidance.

Tips for Sustaining a Balanced pH Diet

Prioritize Fresh Produce: Fill your plate with a variety of alkalizing fruits and vegetables to ensure a rich intake of essential nutrients and antioxidants.

Mindful Meal Planning: Plan your meals ahead, focusing on creating well-balanced combinations of alkaline ingredients to maintain pH equilibrium.

Hydration is Key: Stay adequately hydrated with alkaline beverages like water with lemon or herbal teas to support detoxification and pH balance.

Limit Acidic Beverages: Reduce consumption of acidic beverages like coffee, soda, and alcohol to minimize acidity in the body.

Opt for Plant-Based Proteins: Incorporate plant-based protein sources like legumes, tofu, and quinoa for alkaline-rich nourishment.

Embrace Healthy Fats: Choose alkalizing fats such as avocados, nuts, and olive oil to support cellular health and balance inflammation.

Monitor Acid-Forming Foods: Limit processed foods, refined sugars, and animal products to maintain an alkaline-friendly diet.

Alkaline Snacking: Opt for alkaline-rich snacks like fresh fruits, raw veggies with hummus, or almond butter on rice cakes.

Consider pH-Testing: Use pH test strips to monitor your body's pH levels periodically and adjust your diet accordingly.

Mind Your Stress: Manage stress through practices like meditation, yoga, or deep breathing, as stress can impact the body's acidity.

Remember, sustaining a balanced pH diet is a lifestyle commitment that fosters improved energy levels, supports immune function, and promotes overall well-being. By incorporating these professional tips into your daily routine, you can empower yourself to lead a healthier and more alkaline life.

Acknowledgments

We would like to express our sincere appreciation to everyone who helped create this thorough information on the acid-alkaline diet.

We would like to thank the hardworking group of nutritionists, dietitians, and health professionals who contributed their knowledge and thoughts. Their in-depth expertise and dedication to holistic well-being have greatly influenced this resource.

Special thanks go out to the talented chefs who created the delicious recipes included in this manual. Their inventiveness and culinary prowess have added to the allure of adopting an acid-alkaline lifestyle.

We are also appreciative of the scientists and researchers whose work opened the path for a better comprehension of the effects of the Acid-Alkaline Diet on health. Their ground-breaking research has greatly influenced our strategy.

We want to thank our readers and followers for their steadfast support. Your zeal and enquisitiveness motivate us to carry out our goal of advancing wellbeing via nourishing knowledge.

Together, we are dedicated to educating others about the benefits of an acid-alkaline diet and lifestyle so that you may live a life filled with vigor, balance, and long-lasting health. We appreciate your participation in this enlightening journey.

Bonus 20 Days Meal Plan

Day 1:

- ❖ **Breakfast:** Green smoothie with spinach, banana, kiwi, and almond milk
- ❖ **Lunch:** Lentil and vegetable salad with lemon-tahini dressing
- ❖ **Snack:** Sliced cucumber and hummus
- ❖ **Dinner:** Grilled portobello mushrooms with quinoa and steamed asparagus

Day 2:

- ❖ **Breakfast:** Oatmeal topped with mixed berries and chopped almonds
- ❖ **Lunch:** Mixed greens salad with grilled tofu, bell peppers, and balsamic vinaigrette
- ❖ **Snack:** Carrot and celery sticks with almond butter
- ❖ **Dinner:** Baked salmon with roasted Brussels sprouts and quinoa

Day 3:

- ❖ **Breakfast:** Chia seed pudding with coconut milk, topped with sliced mango
- ❖ **Lunch:** Zucchini noodles with tomato sauce and chickpeas
- ❖ **Snack:** Handful of mixed nuts
- ❖ **Dinner:** Stir-fried tempeh with broccoli, bell peppers, and brown rice

Day 4:

- ❖ **Breakfast:** Greek yogurt with fresh berries and a drizzle of honey
- ❖ **Lunch:** Spinach and avocado wrap with hummus
- ❖ **Snack:** Apple slices with almond butter
- ❖ **Dinner:** Stuffed bell peppers with quinoa, black beans, and salsa

Day 5:

- ❖ **Breakfast:** Scrambled eggs with sautéed spinach and cherry tomatoes
- ❖ **Lunch:** Cauliflower rice stir-fry with mixed vegetables and tofu
- ❖ **Snack:** Rice cakes with sliced avocado
- ❖ **Dinner:** Baked sweet potato with black bean and corn salsa

Day 6:

- ❖ **Breakfast:** Smoothie bowl with mixed berries, banana, almond milk, and a sprinkle of chia seeds
- ❖ **Lunch:** Quinoa and black bean salad with diced avocado and lime-cilantro dressing
- ❖ **Snack:** Rice crackers with guacamole
- ❖ **Dinner:** Grilled vegetable platter with a side of hummus

Day 7:

- ❖ **Breakfast:** Overnight oats with almond milk, sliced peaches, and a touch of cinnamon

* **Lunch:** Spinach and arugula salad with grilled tempeh, walnuts, and raspberry vinaigrette
* **Snack:** Celery sticks with almond butter
* **Dinner:** Baked cod with herbed quinoa and steamed broccoli

Day 8:

* **Breakfast:** Scrambled tofu with sautéed mushrooms, bell peppers, and spinach
* **Lunch:** Lentil soup with a side of mixed greens and lemon-tahini dressing
* **Snack:** Mixed fruit bowl (pineapple, melon, berries)
* **Dinner:** Stuffed acorn squash with wild rice, cranberries, and pecans

Day 9:

* **Breakfast:** Whole grain toast topped with sliced avocado and cherry tomatoes
* **Lunch:** Chickpea and vegetable stir-fry with sesame-ginger sauce
* **Snack:** Handful of almonds and dried apricots
* **Dinner:** Grilled eggplant rolls stuffed with quinoa and roasted red pepper

Day 10:

* **Breakfast:** Acai bowl with granola, coconut flakes, and mixed fruit
* **Lunch:** Cabbage and carrot slaw with grilled portobello mushrooms and a light vinaigrette

❖ **Snack:** Sliced pear with cashew butter

❖ **Dinner:** Spaghetti squash with marinara sauce and a side of steamed green beans

Day 11:

❖ **Breakfast:** Banana walnut smoothie with almond milk and a dash of cinnamon

❖ **Lunch:** Spinach and quinoa salad with roasted beets, goat cheese, and balsamic vinaigrette

❖ **Snack:** Baby carrots with hummus

❖ **Dinner:** Baked tempeh with sweet potato mash and steamed broccoli

Day 12:

❖ **Breakfast:** Chia seed pudding with almond milk, topped with sliced kiwi and shredded coconut

❖ **Lunch:** Mixed greens with grilled tofu, cherry tomatoes, cucumber, and a lemon-tahini dressing

❖ **Snack:** Rice cakes with almond butter and sliced strawberries

❖ **Dinner:** Stuffed zucchini boats with quinoa, black beans, and salsa

Day 13:

❖ **Breakfast:** Greek yogurt parfait with mixed berries, honey, and crushed nuts

* **Lunch:** Brown rice bowl with sautéed mixed vegetables and a drizzle of teriyaki sauce
* **Snack:** Mixed nuts and dried cranberries
* **Dinner:** Grilled portobello mushroom burger on a whole grain bun with a side salad

Day 14:

* **Breakfast:** Omelette with spinach, bell peppers, and feta cheese
* **Lunch:** Lentil and vegetable stew with a side of whole grain bread
* **Snack:** Apple slices with peanut butter
* **Dinner:** Baked salmon with quinoa and steamed asparagus

Day 15:

* **Breakfast:** Smoothie with pineapple, mango, spinach, and coconut water
* **Lunch:** Chickpea and avocado wrap with mixed greens and a lemon-tahini dressing
* **Snack:** Rice crackers with guacamole and salsa
* **Dinner:** Stir-fried tofu with broccoli, bell peppers, and brown rice

Day 16:

* **Breakfast:** Acai smoothie bowl with granola, sliced banana, and a drizzle of honey

- ❖ **Lunch:** Quinoa salad with roasted vegetables, chickpeas, and a balsamic vinaigrette
- ❖ **Snack:** Sliced cucumber with hummus
- ❖ **Dinner:** Baked cod with quinoa and sautéed spinach

Day 17:

- ❖ **Breakfast:** Greek yogurt with mixed berries, chia seeds, and a sprinkle of cinnamon
- ❖ **Lunch:** Spinach and arugula salad with grilled tempeh, walnuts, and a raspberry vinaigrette
- ❖ **Snack:** Almonds and dried apricots
- ❖ **Dinner:** Stuffed bell peppers with quinoa, black beans, and a tomato-herb sauce

Day 18:

- ❖ **Breakfast:** Whole grain toast topped with smashed avocado and cherry tomatoes
- ❖ **Lunch:** Lentil soup with a side of mixed greens and lemon-tahini dressing
- ❖ **Snack:** Mixed fruit bowl (pineapple, melon, berries)
- ❖ **Dinner:** Grilled eggplant slices with quinoa tabbouleh

Day 19:

- ❖ **Breakfast:** Chia seed pudding with almond milk, topped with sliced peaches and chopped nuts

- ❖ **Lunch:** Chickpea and vegetable stir-fry with sesame-ginger sauce
- ❖ **Snack:** Rice cakes with almond butter and sliced pear
- ❖ **Dinner:** Baked sweet potato with black bean and corn salsa

Day 20:

- ❖ **Breakfast:** Scrambled eggs with sautéed spinach, bell peppers, and a touch of feta cheese
- ❖ **Lunch:** Mixed greens with grilled tofu, cucumber, and a lemon-tahini dressing
- ❖ **Snack:** Carrot and celery sticks with hummus
- ❖ **Dinner:** Grilled portobello mushrooms with quinoa and steamed asparagus

Congratulations on completing this 20-day journey of nourishing meals aligned with the Acid-Alkaline Diet. By following this meal plan, you've nurtured your body with alkalizing ingredients, embraced a variety of flavors, and supported your overall well-being. Remember that this is just the beginning of your continued commitment to a balanced and healthful lifestyle. Feel free to repeat the plan or use it as inspiration to create your own alkaline-focused meals for sustained vitality and optimal health.